Aya Chakroun
Intissar Helali

Myelogram in macrophage activation syndrome

Aya Chakroun
Intissar Helali

Myelogram in macrophage activation syndrome

Search for new predictive criteria for the diagnosis of secondary MAS in adults

ScienciaScripts

Imprint
Any brand names and product names mentioned in this book are subject to trademark, brand or patent protection and are trademarks or registered trademarks of their respective holders. The use of brand names, product names, common names, trade names, product descriptions etc. even without a particular marking in this work is in no way to be construed to mean that such names may be regarded as unrestricted in respect of trademark and brand protection legislation and could thus be used by anyone.

Cover image: www.ingimage.com

This book is a translation from the original published under ISBN 978-620-3-41248-2.

Publisher:
Sciencia Scripts
is a trademark of
Dodo Books Indian Ocean Ltd., member of the OmniScriptum S.R.L Publishing group
str. A.Russo 15, of. 61, Chisinau-2068, Republic of Moldova Europe
Printed at: see last page
ISBN: 978-620-3-68573-2

TABLE OF CONTENTS

INTRODUCTION..7

PATIENTS AND METHODS...10

I-Patients 11

I-1 Inclusion criteria : 11

I-3 Exclusion criteria : 11

II Methods : 11

II.1 - Data collection 11

II.1.1- Data collection methods : 11

II.1.2- Parameters studied : 12

II.1.2.1- Demographic and clinical characteristics :......................12

II.1.2.2- Biological parameters : 12

II.1.2.3- Cytological parameters : 13

II.1.2.4- Other parameters : 14

II-3- Division into two groups SAM / non SAM : 15

III- Statistical analysis : 15

IV- Bibliographic research : 15

V- Declaration of interest : 16

VI- Ethical considerations : 16

RESULTS..17

I- General data Study population :...18

II- Demographic, clinical and cytological characteristics of the patients included in the two groups "SAM" and "Non SAM" :...........................19

II-1 Demographic characteristics of the two groups : 19

II-2 Clinical and evolutionary characteristics of the two groups : 20

II-3 Biological characteristics of the two groups : 24

Blood Count : 24

Ferritinemia : 25

Triglyceridemia : 25

Fibrinogenemia : 25

- Transaminases : 26

Bilirubinemia : 26

PAL :..26

Gamma-GT : 26

LDH : 26

- Natremia : 27

CRP : 27

- Albuminemia : 27

II-4. Cytological characteristics of both groups : Data on the first diagnostic reading 29

III. Searching for cytological criteria to optimise the diagnosis of secondary MAS in adults..31

III.1-The richness of the marrow : 31

III.2-The number of macrophages per 1000 nucleated elements : 31

III.3-Hemophagocytosis images : 32

III-4 The nature of the phagocytosed elements : 32

III-5 Images of multiple haemophagocytosis : 33

IV- Search for a predictive model of MAS diagnosis 35

DISCUSSION 38

I- Impact of demographic parameters on the diagnosis of MAS :........40

II- Impact of clinical parameters in the diagnosis of MAS : 42

III-Impact of biological parameters in diagnostic orientation :..........43

IV- Contribution of the myelogram study in the diagnosis of MAS: interest of the research of new cytological parameters.....................45

CONCLUSION 49

REFERENCES 52

ANNEXES 58

LIST OF FIGURES

Figure 1: Flow chart of the study population 18

Figure 2: Distribution of the 35 patients according to department of origin 19

Figure 3: Age distribution of the two groups 20

Figure 4: Main pathologies causing MAS 22

Figure 5: ROC curves for biochemical parameters associated with the diagnosis of MAS 29

Figure 6: Marrow richness at 2nd reading 31

Figure 7: ROC curves for the two regression models 37

LIST OF TABLES

Table N° 1: Demographic, clinical and evolutionary characteristics of the patients included in the two groups 23

Table 2: Summary of CBC data in both groups 24

Table 3: Characteristics of the biological parameters in the two groups 28

Table 4: Cytological characteristics of the first diagnostic reading 30

Table 5: Grading of haemophagocytosis intensity in the two groups.32

Table 6: Cytological characteristics of the second reading 33

Table 7: Intensity of haemophagocytosis and cytopenias 34

Table 8: Intensity of haemophagocytosis and hyperferritinemia in SAM patients..35

Table 9: Intensity of haemophagocytosis and hyperferritinemia in "non MAS" patients..35

Table 10: Equations/models for predicting MAS diagnosis.................36

Table 11: Characteristics of the regression equations 36

INTRODUCTION

Macrophage activation syndrome (MAS) or haemophagocytic lymphohistiocytosis (HLH) is a hyperinflammatory condition characterised by non-specific and uncontrolled activation of the monocyte-macrophage system. The syndrome involves benign tissue proliferation of histiocytes/macrophages with uncontrolled haemophagocytic activity. It is a severe disease with a poor prognosis, often fatal if not treated promptly. HLH is a rare disease [1,2].

There are two main nosological frameworks:

- Primary MAS, affecting mainly children. Also called familial HLH, this category is conditioned by genetic abnormalities in the process of cellular cytotoxicity.
- Secondary MAS occurs at any age but mainly in adults. Still called acquired or secondary HLH, this category is associated with infections, haematological malignancies, autoimmune diseases, etc. The treatment in this case is mainly etiological.

MAS is a rare condition whose prevalence is probably underestimated due to its diagnostic difficulty [2,3].

Indeed, there is no pathognomonic sign or biological test specific to MAS. Thus, in practice, the diagnosis is made when there is a suggestive combination of clinical, biological and cytological arguments, which are certainly not specific.

Nevertheless, cytology plays a major role in the diagnosis of this disease. Thus, the bone marrow smear aims not only to look for images of haemophagocytosis but also for a possible underlying etiology.

Haemophagocytosis is a criterion included in various diagnostic scores for MAS, including the HLH-2004 [4] and the H-Score [5]. In the latter score, haemophagocytosis was given a high weighting. However, the image of haemophagocytosis is not specific to MAS. Indeed, it can be found in other situations of cytokine overload such as in severe sepsis or post-transfusion.

In contrast, the absence of haemophagocytosis images does not rule out the diagnosis. In addition, few studies have examined the qualitative study of the myelogram and the cyto-morphological features observed in MAS [6,7].

In this regard, to the best of our knowledge, theliterature does not define consensus requirements regarding the number of threshold images to be observed or the type of phagocytic cells, as criteria that could improve the sensitivity of orientation towards the positive diagnosis.

We therefore conducted a prospective study including all cases of suspected secondary HLH presented for myelogram at the haematology department of La Rabta Hospital over a period of 20 months, from June 2017 to January 2019.

The objectives of our study were to:

- Describe the clinical, biological and cytological characteristics of patients with a suspected diagnosis of secondary MAS.
- To search for quantitative and qualitative cytological criteria to optimise the diagnostic orientation towards the diagnosis of secondary MAS (HLH) in adults.

PATIENTS AND METHODS

I-Patients

We conducted a prospective single-centre evaluative study that collected all cases of suspected macrophagic activation syndrome (MAS/secondary HLH) in adults presented to the haematology department of the CHU la Rabta in order to perform a myelogram during the period from June 2017 to January 2019.

I-1 Inclusion criteria :

We included in the study :

- All adult cases, over 16 years of age, in whom the diagnosis of MAS was suspected by the medical team in charge of the patient.

I-2 Criteria for non-inclusion :

The following were not included in our study

- Children's MAS

- Patients who were missing more than three data items necessary to retain the diagnosis.

I-3 Exclusion criteria :

- Patients who had not undergone sternal puncture.

- Patients whose 2nd smear reading could not be performed due to :

    Unavailability of reserve (unstained) slides. (2nd reading done on slides different from those used for the 1st diagnostic reading)

    Hemodiluted or uninterpretable spare blades

II Methods :

II.1 - Data collection

II.1.1- Data collection methods :

Epidemiological, clinical and para-clinical data were collected using a data sheet (Appendix 1) prepared by a haematologist biologist and validated by the head of the haematology department. This form was completed for each patient at the time of suspected diagnosis of MAS either by the attending physician or by the haematology resident conducting the study.

II.1.2- Parameters studied :

II.1.2.1- Demographic and clinical characteristics :

Data on demographic characteristics included age at diagnosis, gender, department of origin, and personal medical and surgical history.

Data on clinical characteristics included:

immunosuppressive terrain (HIV infection, immunosuppressive therapy and corticosteroid therapy)

the maximum temperature

the presence of organomegaly (splenomegaly, hepatomegaly, adenopathy)

skin, lung or neurological manifestations

the final diagnosis chosen by the medical team in charge of the patient in question (SAM/ non SAM)

The selected etiology of MAS and the evolution of the

II.1.2.2- Biological parameters :

When the diagnosis of MAS was suspected, the results of the following tests were noted. It should be noted that any missing biological tests were systematically indicated. Thus, the parameters collected were :

Blood count, Ferritinemia, Triglyceridemia, Fibrinogenemia, Lactate dehydrogenase (LDH), Natremia, Aspartame Aminotransferase (AST or SGOT), Alanine Aminotransferase (ALAT or SGPT), Total bilirubinemia, Alkaline phosphatase (ALP), Gamma glutamyl transferase (GammaGT), C-Reactive Protein (CRP) and Albuminemia

II.1.2.3- Cytological parameters :

<u>The first reading</u> :

A bone marrow smear at the time of suspected diagnosis of MAS was performed in the patients. Sternal puncture or bone marrow biopsy (with BOM impression) was performed as indicated by the patient's physician.

After staining with May Grunwald and Giemsa (MGG), this cytological study is organised in two stages:

> 1st stage: a study at low magnification (x10) with the main objective, in our study, of estimating the medullary richness.

Thus, after examination of several fields, the richness of the marrow is estimated by a semi-quantitative rating (from 0 to ++++). A deserted marrow is rated 0, a poor marrow (+), a moderately rich marrow (++), a marrow of normal richness (+++) and a very rich marrow (++++).

> 2nd stage: a study at high magnification (x100), involving 200 to 500 cells examined. The main purpose of this reading was to record data concerning the presence or absence of macrophages, the presence or absence of haemophagocytosis images and any elements in favour of the aetiology: leishmanias, suspect cells, etc.

<u>The second reading</u> :

This is a more detailed reading of the myelograms, carried out at the end of the period of collection of all data (i.e. from June 2019). This reading was carried out in a single-blind manner, by a trained cytologist, and concerned slides different from those used for the [1st] reading, which were archived. Thus, among the unstained reserve slides, the richest slides were studied.

The collected slides were stained with May Grunwald and Giemsa (MGG). Then, the cytological study was organised in two steps, as previously described, but a larger number of cells (1000 nucleated elements) was examined.

The objectives of this reading were to clarify :

- The number of macrophages/1000 nuclei

- Intensity of haemophagocytosis: the number of haemophagocytosis images observed/ 1000 nucleated elements

- the nature of the elements phagocytosed

- as well as the presence of multiple phagocytosis images.

❖ An image of haemophagocytosis is defined by the observation of a macrophage that has phagocytosed one or more figured elements.

❖ An image of multiple haemophagocytosis is arbitrarily defined as a macrophage having phagocytosed more than two figured elements (Appendix 2).

❖ The intensity of haemophagocytosis is arbitrarily graded as follows:

Grade I: 1-3 images of haemophagocytosis

Grade II: 4-6 images of haemophagocytosis

Grade III: 7-10 images of haemophagocytosis

Grade IV: >10 images of haemophagocytosis

All these data were collected by means of a cytological form (Appendix 3)

II.1.2.4- Other parameters :

In the search for evidence in favour of the possible aetiology of MAS, the results of the following para-clinical investigations were also recorded:

Cytobacteriological examination of urine (ECBU), Blood cultures, Viral serologies: HIV, CMV, EBV, hepatitis B and C, Culture of other biological products, Osteo-medullary biopsy (BOM), Chest X-ray, Computed tomography (CT)

II-3- Division into two groups SAM / non SAM :

All suspected SAM cases were divided into two groups after consultation of the medical records at the end of the patient inclusion period (i.e. January 2019): "SAM group" and "non SAM group".

Thus, the "SAM group" includes patients whose positive diagnosis has been retained by the medical team in charge of the patient on the basis of clinico-biological arguments and clearly recorded in the medical file and the patient treated accordingly.

 The "non-SAM group" includes cases where the medical team in charge of the patient has not retained this diagnosis.

III- Statistical analysis :

All demographic, clinical, biological and score data were entered into Microsoft Excel 2010. Statistical analysis was performed using SPSS 25.0 software.

A test of the normality of the distribution of the different parameters studied was provided by the Shapiro test and the Kolmogorov-Smirnov test.

For qualitative variables, numbers and relative frequencies (percentages) were expressed. For quantitative variables, means and standard deviations or medians and extremes after checking the normality of the distributions.

Comparisons of percentages on independent series were made using the Pearson chi-square test. In case of invalidity of this test, the two-tailed Fisher exact test was used. The comparison of quantitative variables was carried out by the Student's T-test for variables with a normal distribution and by the non-parametric Mann-Whitney test where appropriate.

For all tests, a *p-value of* <0.05 was used to conclude that there was a statistically significant difference.

IV- Bibliographic research :

The bibliographic references were collected by EndNote X7 software from :

PubMed

ScienceDirect

EM consults

The keywords used for the search were: macrophage activation syndrome, myelogram, secondary HLH, hemophagocytosis, Macrophage activation syndrome, diagnosis, adult.

V- Declaration of interest :

We, the author and supervisor, declare that we have no conflict of interest in relation to this work.

VI- Ethical considerations :

This study did not raise any ethical issues that would have warranted approval by the local ethics committee of our institution. All the tests performed were deliberately prescribed by the doctors in charge of the patients included during their hospitalisation and the parameters studied were obtained without any additional cost. The confidentiality of the patients' identities and the information collected was respected.

RESULTS

I- General data Study population :

During the inclusion period, 54 suspected cases of MAS were identified. Nineteen subjects were excluded from the study (in 11 cases a sternal puncture was not performed, in 3 cases spare (unstained) slides were not available and in 5 cases the slides found were either hemodiluted or uninterpretable).

In the end, thirty-five cases were selected. They were divided into two groups "SAM group" and "non SAM group" according to whether the final diagnosis was retained by the team in charge or not. (Figure 1).

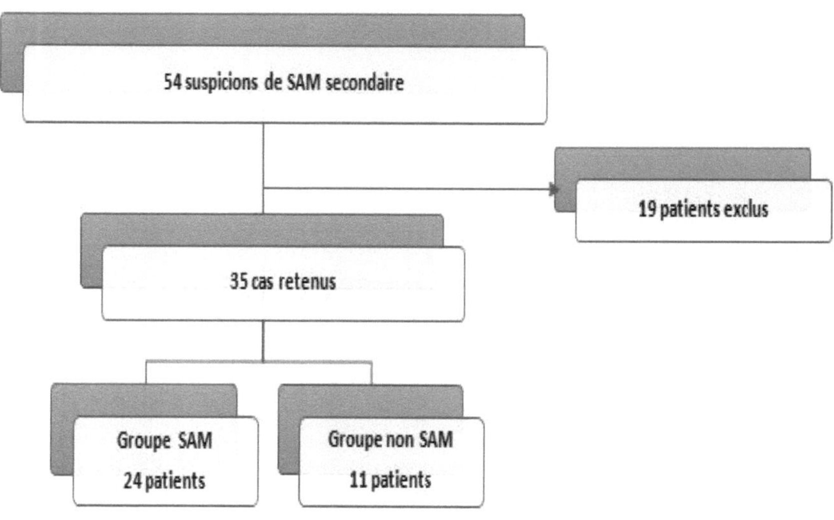

Figure 1: Flow chart of the study population

In the 35 patients suspected of having MAS, the sex ratio was 0.95. The median age was 45.47 years with extremes ranging from 17 to 80 years.

The majority of patients came from a medical service (92%, n=32) and only three from surgical services (Figure 2).

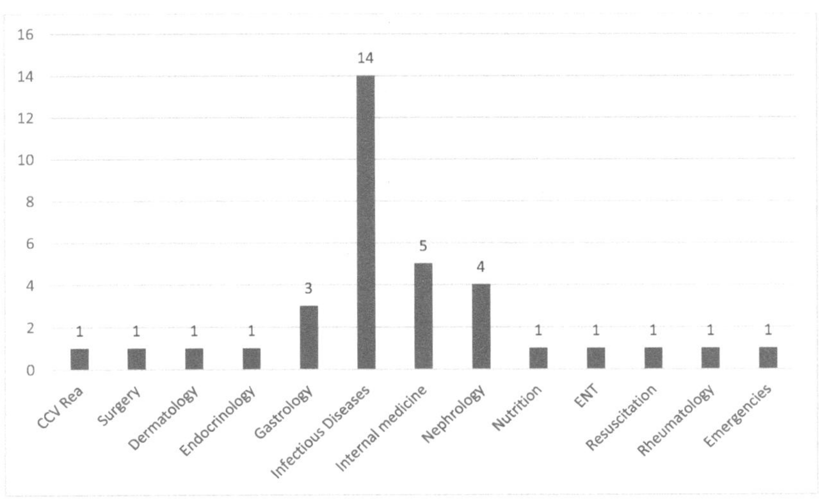

Figure 2: Distribution of the 35 patients according to department of origin

II- Demographic, clinical and cytological characteristics of the patients included in the two groups "SAM" and "Non SAM":

II-1 Demographic characteristics of the two groups :

In the SAM group, women predominated (sex ratio=0.72). In the "non-SAM group", men represented 64% of the subjects, i.e. a sex ratio of 1.75.

However, there was no statistically significant difference in gender between the two groups (p=0.227).

Patients in the "non-SAM group" were significantly older than those in the "SAM group" (respectively mean age ± standard deviation in the "non-SAM group" = 53 years± 14.82 versus 42 years± 17.25; p=0.036).

Figure 3 shows the age distribution of patients and controls respectively.

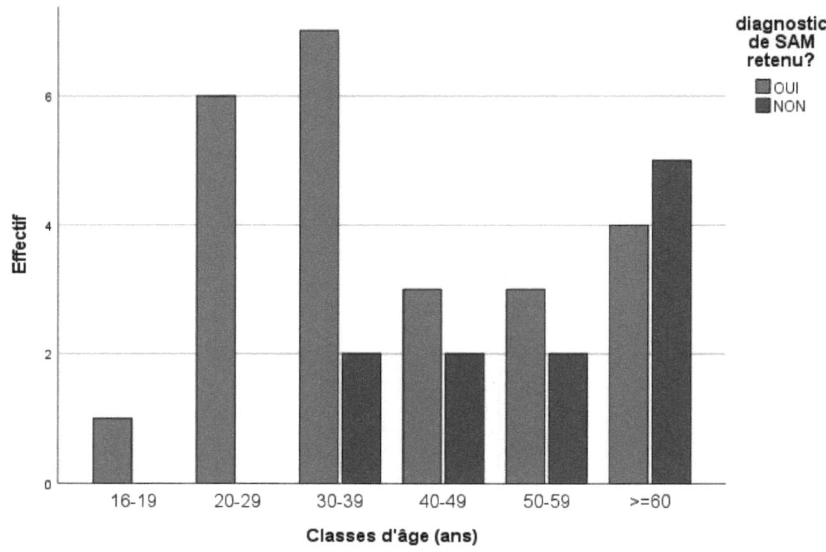

Figure 3: Age distribution of the two groups

Almost all SAM patients came from a medical ward (23/24). And almost half (10/24) were hospitalised in the infectious diseases department

In the "non-SAM group", 9 patients were from a medical ward and 2 patients were hospitalised in a surgical ward (surgery and ENT).

II-2 Clinical and evolutionary characteristics of the two groups:

The immune status of patients was recorded and was comparable between the two groups (p=0.721).

In the "SAM group", 15 subjects (63%) were immunocompromised (4 with HIV, 4 on corticosteroid therapy and 7 on one or more immunosuppressive treatments).

In the "non-SAM group", 6 subjects were immunocompromised, two of whom had HIV.

The main clinical signs described during MAS were studied in both groups.

Concerning fever, the median temperature of the subjects in the "SAM group" was significantly higher than that observed in the "non-SAM group" (i.e. 39.55°C [36.5°C - 41°C] in the SAM group versus 38.7°C [37°C - 41°C] in the "non-SAM group"; p=0.006)

It is noteworthy that the majority of patients with a successful diagnosis (22/24) in the SAM group had a temperature ≥39°C compared to five in the non-SAM group.

Regarding the presence of organomegaly, six subjects in the "SAM group" had splenomegaly or hepatomegaly and five patients had both hepatomegaly and splenomegaly.

In the "no MAS group", almost half of the subjects had splenomegaly or hepatomegaly and three had hepatosplenomegaly.

However, we could not find any statistically significant difference between the two groups (p=0.263 and p=0.685). (Table 1)

The presence of superficial or deep adenopathy was more frequent in the SAM group (n=8 versus n=2 in the Non SAM group) without any statistically significant difference (p= 0, 447).

The skin manifestations were mainly rash and purpura, and their presence was comparable in both groups, p=1.

The respiratory manifestations were cough, haemoptysis, dyspnoea and pleurisy. These signs were often associated. In both groups, almost half of the subjects had respiratory manifestations, p=0.721.

The neurological signs were mainly confusion and temporo-spatial disorientation. These disorders were more frequently encountered in the

SAM group, but were not a discriminating factor between the two groups. (p=0,387)

After a series of investigations, an aetiology for MAS was found in 22 patients. The main aetiologies found were infectious diseases, systemic diseases, neoplasia and drug-related causes (figure 4)

Infectious causes were the most frequent (54% of the patients in the "SAM group"), of which 5 patients had active tuberculosis.

Figure 4 shows the distribution of patients according to the selected causal pathology.

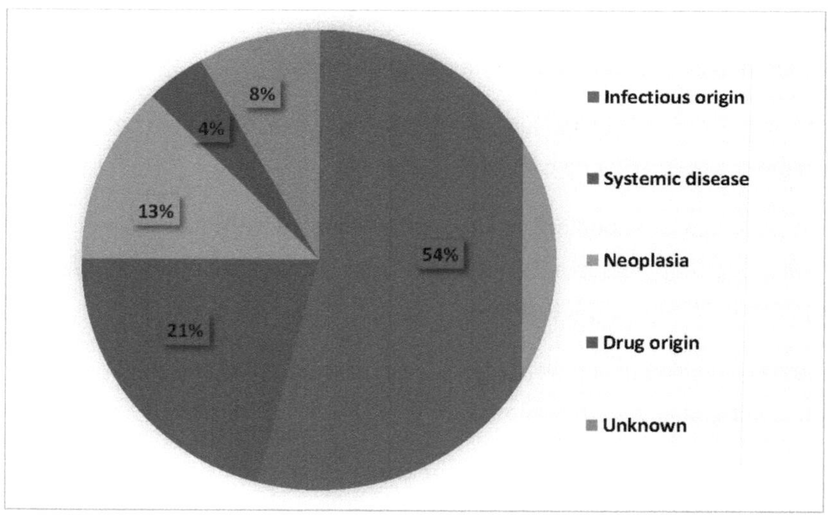

Figure 4: Main pathologies causing MAS

Table 1 summarises the demographic, clinical and developmental characteristics of the patients included in the two groups

Table N° 1: Demographic, clinical and evolutionary characteristics of the patients included in the two groups

Clinical features	SAM Group (n=24)	Non-SAM group (n=11)	p
	n (%)	n (%)	
Sex-ratio (Men/ Women)	0,72	1,75	0,227
Average age (years), standard deviation	42 ±17,25	53±14,82	**0,036**
Median temperature, extremes	39,55°C 36.5°C-41°C].	38,7°C 37°C - 41°C]	**0,006**
Fever			
<38°C	1 (4%)	5 (45%)	**0,007**
≥38°C	23 (96%)	6 (55%)	
Hepatomegaly alone	6(25%)	5(45%)	0,263
Splenomegaly alone	10 (42%)	6 (55%)	0,478
Hepato splenomegaly	5 (21%)	3 (27%)	0,685
Adenopathies	8 (33%)	2 (18%)	0,447
Skin manifestations	5 (21%)	2(18%)	1
Respiratory manifestations	11 (46%)	4 (36%)	0,721
Neurological manifestations	7 (29%)	1(9%)	0,387
Evolution			
Number of deaths	9 (37,5%)	1 (9%)	0,12
Early death (< 1 month)	7 (29%)	1 (9%)	0,38

In sum, among the demographic and clinical parameters, age and fever appeared to be discriminating factors between the two groups.

II-3 Biological characteristics of the two groups :

<u>Blood Count</u> :

The CBC data in both groups are summarised in Table 2

Table 1: Summary of CBC data in the two groups

Parameters	SAM group (n=24) Median [inf-sup].	Non-SAM group (n=11) Median [inf-sup].	p
Leukocytes(/mm3)	3390 [450 -18 990]	4640 [850 -15120]	0,93
PNN (/mm3)	2375 [20 - 16400]	2980 [0 - 12680]	0,903
Lymphocytes(/mm3)	485 [170 - 2760]	1090 [240 - 1950]	0,198
Monocytes (/mm3)	310 [20 - 2900]	490 [10 - 2170]	0,72
Hemoglobin (g/dL)	6.85 [2,1-12,6]	5,4 [4,2-10,9]	0,283
Platelets (/mm3)	75000 [3000 -332 000]	58 000 [11 000- 189 000]	0,54

Leukopenia (WBC<4000/mm3) was a common haematological finding in both groups. Indeed, n=13 in the "SAM group" vs n=5 in the "non SAM group". At the same time, neutropenia (<1500/mm3) was observed in 11 patients with MAS vs. 5 in the "non MAS group".

Thrombocytopenia was by far the most frequently observed haematological disorder. Indeed, ¾ of the patients with MAS and almost all of the patients in the "non-ASM group" (91%) were thrombocytopenic at the time of suspected diagnosis.

However, no CBC parameter was significantly associated with the diagnosis of MAS.

<u>Ferritinemia :</u>

The median ferritin level was significantly higher in the SAM group than in the Non SAM group (4023 µg/L [498 µg/L - 51231 µg/L] in the SAM group versus 1168 µg/L [24 µg/L - 4935 µg/L] in the Non SAM group, respectively; p=0.04). (Table 3).

Hyperferritinemia of more than 3000 µg/L was found in 62.5% of MAS patients vs. 20% of non-ASM patients, p= 0.024.

In contrast, severe hyperferritinaemia (>10,000 µg/L) was observed in only seven patients with MAS. No patient in the "non-ASM group" had severe hyperferritinemia.

<u>Triglyceridemia :</u>

The median triglyceride value was significantly higher in patients with MAS than in the "non-ASM group" (respectively; 3.37 mmol/L vs. 1.2 mmol/L; p=0.000). (Table 3)

Hypertriglyceridaemia of more than 4 mmol/L was observed in ten MAS patients (42%). No patient in the "non-ASM group" had such a level.

<u>Fibrinogenemia :</u>

Fibrinogen measurements were performed in 14 patients in the SAM group and 7 in the non-SAM group. The median values in the two groups were comparable (3.66 g/L [2 g/L-8.11 g/L] versus 3.59 g/L [2.24-6.29] in the "non-SAM group; p=0.971). (Table 3)

- Transaminases :

The median SGOT value was lower in MAS patients than in non-ASM patients, but no statistical association was demonstrated (37.5 U/L [6 U/L; 1035U/L] vs 45 U/L [19U/L; 75U/L]; p=0.93).

The median SGPT value was 21 U/L [6 U/L; 884 U/L] in the "SAM group" and 28.5 U/L [6 U/L-62 U/L] in the "non SAM group". There was no statistically significant difference between the two groups (p=0.971). (Table 3)

Bilirubin :

In the "SAM group", the median bilirubin value was 10 mg/L [1 mg/L - 366 mg/L]. In contrast, in the "non-SAM group" the median bilirubin value was 12 mg/L [3 mg/L - 219.6 mg/L]. The distribution of values for this parameter in the two groups was comparable (p=0.636).

PAL :

There was no statistically significant difference between the two groups (p=1) regarding this parameter. Thus, in the "SAM group", the median PAL value was 100 U/L [23 U/L - 313 U/L]. A comparable distribution of values was observed in the "non-SAM group" (median=96 U/L with [47U/L - 199 U/L]).

Gamma-GT :

This test was performed in 21 patients with MAS in whom the median value was higher than that observed in the "non-ASM group" (respectively, "MAS group" median= 89 U/L [12 U/L to 1114 U/L] versus "non-ASM group", median value= 42 U/L [11U/L; 354U/L]). However, this difference did not reach statistical significance (p=0.347).

LDH :

The median LDH value was statistically higher in the "SAM group" than in the "non-SAM group" (679 U/L [187U/L; 1484U/L] versus 422U/L [163U/L; 1621U/L] respectively; p=0.034)

<u>- Natremia :</u>

The median natraemia value was statistically significantly lower in the 'retained MAS group' than in the 'non-retained MAS group' (130.5 mmol/L [123 mmol/L; 143 mmol/L] and 136 mmol/L [131 mmol/L; 145 mmol/L] respectively; p=0.02).

Hyponatremia was observed in 22 MAS patients vs. five patients in the "non-ASM group", p=0.006.

<u>CRP :</u>

The median CRP value was higher in the "SAM group" (123.35 mg/L [19 mg/L - 436.1 mg/L] versus 77.9 mg/L [0-386.7] respectively).

However, this difference was not statistically significant (p=0.451).

<u>- Albumin levels :</u>

Albumin levels were measured in 19 SAM patients and all "non SAM" patients.

There was no statistically significant difference between the two groups (p=0.42) (Table 3)

Table 3 shows the data from the comparative study between the two groups on biological parameters.

Table 2: Characteristics of biological parameters in the two groups

Parameters	SAM Group N=24	Non SAM Group N=11	P
Ferritinemia (µg/L)	4023 [498 – 51231]	1168 [24 - 4935]	**0,04**
Triglyceridemia (mmol/L)	3,37 [0,78-3,35]	1,2 [0,29-3,35]	**10-3**
Fibrinogenemia (g/L)	3,66 [2 - 8,11]	3,59 [2,24 – 6,29]	0,971
SGOT(U/L)	37,5 [6- 1035]	45 [19 - 75]	0,93
SGPT (U/L)	21 [6 - 884]	28,5 [6-62]	0,971
Bilirubinemia (mg/L)	10 [1 - 366]	12 [3 - 219,6].	0,636
Gamma GT (U/L)	89 [12 - 1114]	42 [11 - 354]	0,347
PAL (U/L)	100 [23 - 313]	96 [47 - 199]	1
LDH (U/L)	679 [187 - 1484]	422 [163 - 1621]	**0,034**
Natraemia (mmol/L)	130,5 [123 -143]	136 [131- 145]	**0,02**
CRP (mg/L)	123,35 [19 - 436,1]	77,9 [0- 386,7]	0,451
Albumin levels (g/L)	29,1 [15,8 - 37,8]	31,6 [18,9 - 38,8]	0,42

In the end, the comparative study showed that hyperferritinemia, hypertriglyceridemia, hyponatremia and elevated LDH levels were discriminating parameters between the two SAM and non-SAM groups. Figure 5 summarises the performance of each parameter.

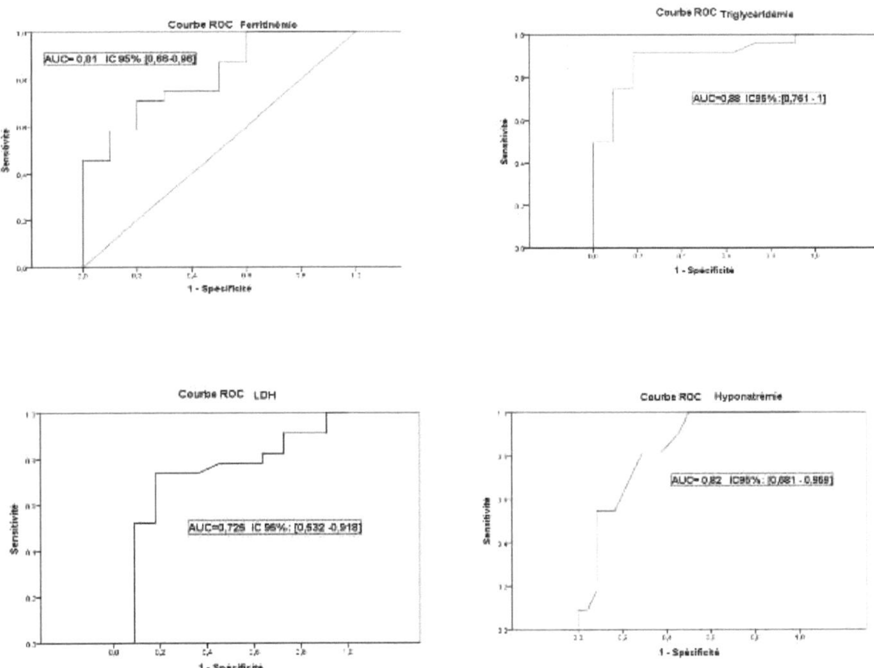

Figure 5: ROC curves for biochemical parameters associated with the diagnosis of MAS

II-4. Cytological characteristics of both groups : Data on the first diagnostic reading

The slide reading at the time of suspected diagnosis of MAS was performed by two experienced cytologists on a number of cells examined between 200 and 500 cells. The final report is validated jointly by the two cytologists.

Table 3: Cytological characteristics of the first diagnostic reading

	"SAM Group n=24	"Non SAM Group N=11	p
	n (%)	n (%)	
Richness of the marrow			0,5
+	0	1(9,1)	
++	8(33,3)	1(9,1)	
+++	9(37,5)	5 (45,5)	
++++	7(29,5)	4 (36,3)	
Presence of macrophages	23 (95,8)	7 (63,6)	**0,02**
Image of haemophagocytosis	18 (75)	5 (45,5)	0,13
Intensity of haemophagocytosis			0,61
A single image	7 (39)	3 (60)	
>an image	11 (61)	2 (40)	

Only the presence of macrophages appears to be associated with the diagnosis of MAS.

III. Search for cytological criteria to optimise the diagnostic orientation towards secondary MAS in adults

III.1-The richness of the marrow :

Marrow richness was estimated at low magnification. Figure 6 summarises the estimated richness of the smears examined in each group.

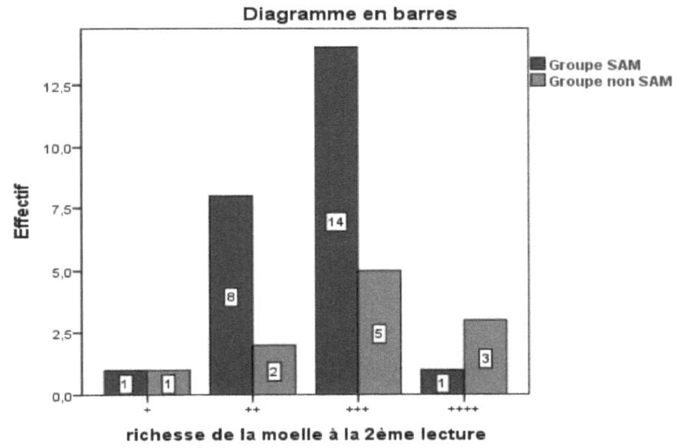

Figure 6: Marrow richness at 2nd reading

The majority of patients in the SAM group (n=22) had moderately rich to rich marrow. However, richer slides were observed in the "non-SAM" group. It should be noted that no desert smears were found. (Figure 6)

III.2-The number of macrophages per 1000 nuclei :

The observation of numerous macrophages was common in both groups. The mean number of macrophages was 26.13/1000 nucleated elements [1-75] in the SAM group and 22.45/1000 nucleated elements [2-48] in the non-SAM group. However, the observed difference was not significant (p=0.588).

Considering the smears that showed a macrophage count of more than 2%, almost half of the slides in both groups were retained.

One third of the slides from the "MAS group" showed a macrophage count of more than 3% compared to four slides from the "non MAS group". And only two slides from MAS patients showed more than 5% macrophage infiltration. This level was not reached in the slides of the other group.

Furthermore, the mean number of macrophages increased with increasing triglyceridaemia: 24.5/1000 cells in patients without hypertriglyceridaemia (n=14) versus 25.7/1000 cells in those with triglyceridaemia >4 mmol/L (n=10).

III.3-Hemophagocytosis images :

The image of haemophagocytosis was found in the majority of the slides studied (63% of the slides in the SAM group vs. 73% of the slides in the non-SAM group).

The intensity of haemophagocytosis was not a discriminating parameter between the groups (p=0.23).

Table 4: Grading of the intensity of haemophagocytosis in the two groups

Intensity of haemophagocytosis	"SAM group n=15	"Non-SAM group n=8	p
Grade I (1-3)	8	6	
Grade II (4-6)	4	2	
Grade III (7-10)	3	0	0,23
Grade IV (>10)	0	0	

III-4 The nature of the phagocytosed elements :

Haemophagocytosis involved all nucleated figurative elements as well as red blood cells (RBC) and platelets (Plq) (Table 6)

Thus, haemophagocytosis of a RBC was found in nine subjects in the "SAM group" compared with three in the "non-SAM group", p=0.4.

Almost half of both groups had platelet haemophagocytosis, p=1.

Erythroblast haemophagocytosis (EB) was found in ten and five subjects in the "SAM group" and "non-SAM group", respectively.

Granule phagocytosis was more frequent in the "SAM group" (60% versus 25% of the "non SAM group", p=0.193.)

Table 5: Cytological characteristics of the second reading

	"SAM group n=24	"Non-SAM group n=11	*p*
	n(%)	n(%)	
Presence of haemophagocytosis images	15 (62,5%)	8 (73%)	0,7
Number of phagocytosed elements/blade (median, extremes)	4 [1-14]	2,5 [1-15]	0,392
GR	1 [0-6]	0 [0-3]	0,265
Plq	0 [0-5]	0,5 [0-9]	0,875
EB	1 [0-7]	1 [0-4]	0,728
Granular	1 [0-3]	0 [0-3]	0,238

III-5 Images of multiple haemophagocytosis :

Images of haemophagocytosis were also looked for and phagocytic cells were identified (Table 7).

These multiple images were encountered in 60% of the subjects in the "SAM group" and 50% in the "non SAM group", p=0.685.

Considering only multiple phagocytosis of nucleated elements, these images were found in 33% of the subjects in the "SAM group" and in 25% of the subjects in the "non SAM group", p=1.

Only two patients in the "SAM group" had more than one image of multiple haemophagocytosis. However, this difference was not significant, p=0.5.

We also assessed the importance of biological disturbances according to the intensity of haemophagocytosis, but we did not find a statistically significant relationship between biological parameters and the number of haemophagocytosis images (p=0.7 "SAM group" and p= 0.12 "non SAM group").

Table 6: Intensity of haemophagocytosis and cytopenias

Intensity of haemophagocytosis	Number of cytopenias			
	No n	Monocytopenia n	Bicytopenia n	Pancytopenia n
	SAM/non SAM	SAM/non SAM	SAM/non SAM	SAM/non SAM
I	0/0	2/1	4/0	3/5
II	1/0	0/0	0/0	3/5
III	0/0	1/0	0/0	1/0

We did not find an association between the intensity of haemophagocytosis and hyperferritinemia.

Table 7: Intensity of haemophagocytosis and hyperferritinemia in SAM patients

	Ferritinemia<3000 (µg/L)	Ferritinemia>3000 (µg/L)	P
Intensity of haemophagocytosis	(n)	(n)	0,38
I	4	5	
II	2	2	
III	2	0	

Table 8: Intensity of haemophagocytosis and hyperferritinemia in "non MAS" patients

	Ferritinemia<3000 (µg/L)	Ferritinemia>3000 (µg/L)	P
Intensity of haemophagocytosis	(n)	(n)	0,5
I	4	1	
II	2	0	

IV- Search for a predictive model for the diagnosis of MAS

We performed a multiple logistic regression incorporating the clinical, biological and cytological parameters defined in the study. The data are summarised in Tables 10 and 11 and Figure 7.

Table 9: Equations/models for predicting MAS diagnosis

Models	Logistic regression equations
Model 1	3.323-0.562* Triglyceridemia +0.106*Age - 0.096*Temperature -0.267*Ferritinemia -0.034 *No. of macrophages/1000 items - 0.34 *No. of haemophagocytosis images/1000 items
Model 2	3.335 -0.097* temperature -0.216* ferritinemia-0.576* triglyceridemia -0.026* macrophages/1000 elements +0.144* granule phagocytosis -0.309* HP intensity grade
Model 3	2.076 -0.23*platelets-0.153*ferritinemia-0.571*triglyceridemia-0.298*intensity grade of HP+0.315*presence of granular phagocytosis-0.11*multiple hemophagocytosis-0.115*organomegaly

Table 10: Characteristics of the regression equations

Models	R-two	Significance ANOVA	AUC [95% CI]	COMMENTS
Model 1	0,545	0,04	0,352 [0,108-0,596]	Triglyceridemia: strong effect No. of HP: medium effect
Model 2	0,571	0,027	0,8 [0.492 -1]	Triglyceridemia: strong effect HP intensity grade: medium effect

| **Model 3** | 0,764 | 0,908 | 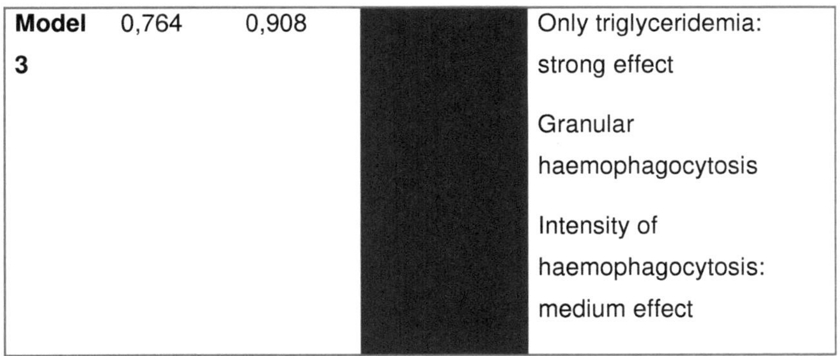 | Only triglyceridemia: strong effect

Granular haemophagocytosis

Intensity of haemophagocytosis: medium effect |

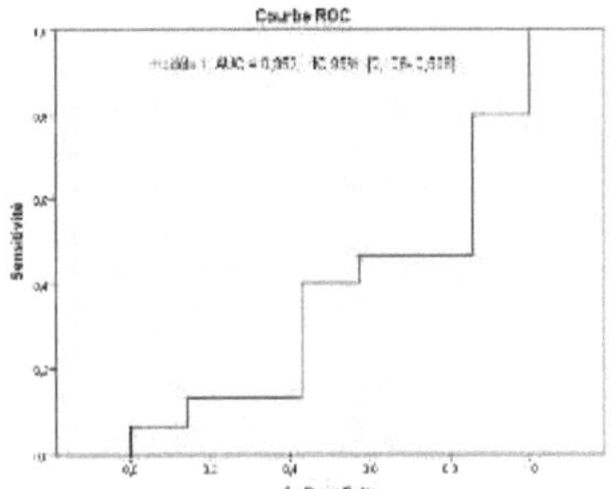
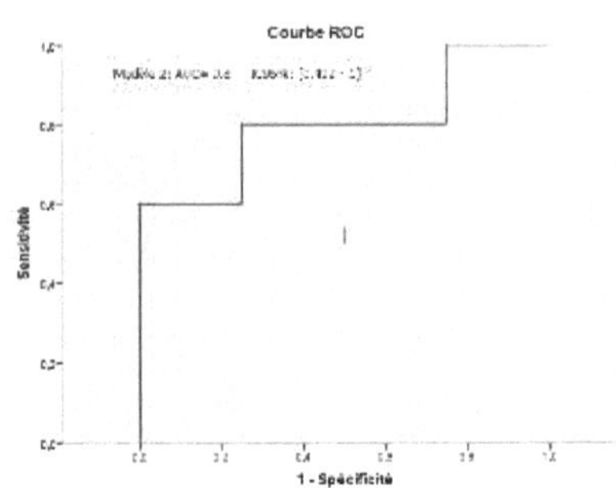

Figure 7: ROC curves for the two regression models

The quality of the three models was moderate (0.54<R-two<0.76). At the same time, these models had low discriminatory power.

The effect attributed to the integration of cytological parameters was small to medium.

Only triglyceride levels appeared to be associated with the diagnosis of MAS in the multivariate study and maintained a strong effect in the decision to diagnose MAS.

DISCUSSION

Macrophage activation syndrome is a condition characterised by excessive stimulation of the immune system leading to systemic inflammation with abnormal phagocytosis of figurative elements and exaggerated release of pro-inflammatory cytokines associated with multi-organ failure [1]. It is a relatively rare entity, but its prevalence is thought to be increasing. Indeed, more than 1500 publications on this topic have appeared since 2004 [2].

In the paediatric setting, the diagnosis of primary MAS is standardised as it is based on the HLH-2004 criteria. However, few national registries for primary MAS exist worldwide [8].

The exact prevalence of secondary MAS in adults remains unknown due to the difficulty in making a positive diagnosis. [2,3]

Indeed, the clinical presentation is very polymorphic, most often associating fever and hepatosplenomegaly. On the biological level, there is no specific test. The association of cytopenia, hyperferritinemia and hypertriglyceridemia should raise the diagnosis and often leads the clinician to perform a myelogram in search of images of haemophagocytosis.

Haemophagocytosis is a criterion included in various diagnostic scores for MAS, including the HLH-2004 for primary MAS [4] and more recently in the H-Score, a new diagnostic score for secondary MAS [5]. In the latter score, haemophagocytosis is given an important weighting.

However, the observation of haemophagocytosis is not specific to MAS. Indeed, it can be found in many other situations such as severe sepsis, autoimmune diseases, with certain drugs or post-transfusion [6].

On the other hand, the absence of haemophagocytosis images does not rule out the diagnosis. Indeed, there are genuine MAS where haemophagocytosis is missing [7].

In addition, few studies have focused on the qualitative study of the myelogram and the cyto-morphological features observed in MAS [6,7].

In this regard, to the best of our knowledge, the literature does not define consensus requirements regarding the number of threshold images to be observed or the type of phagocytic cells, as criteria that could improve the sensitivity of orientation towards the positive diagnosis.

In this prospective study, we first tried to establish the clinical, biological and cytological profile of two groups of "MAS" and "non-ASM" patients, initially suspected of having MAS and presented to the haematology team for a myelogram.

In a second step, we tried to find cytological criteria to optimise the referral to the diagnosis of MAS in adults.

Twenty-four MAS and eleven non-ASM patients were included in the study. We were able to demonstrate a significant association between fever, hyperferritinemia, hypertriglyceridemia, increased LDH and hyponatremia and a positive diagnosis of MAS.

Among the cytological parameters, only the presence of macrophages was associated with the diagnosis of MAS.

In addition, several logistic regression equations explaining the variable "diagnosis of MAS" including parameters from the cytomorphological study were constructed. None showed a significant ability to predict the diagnosis ($0.5 < R2 < 0.75$). The impact of cytological parameters was low to moderate. In contrast, hypertriglyceridaemia was the only parameter with a consistently strong effect ($|\beta| > 0.5$) in retaining the diagnosis.

I- Impact of demographic parameters on the diagnosis of MAS

<u>The genre</u>

In our study, a female predominance was found in the "MAS group" (sex ratio=0.72). The data in the literature are discordant, but the authors agree that gender is not a discriminatory criterion for MAS [9].

Age

The median age of our population was 42 years. This result is consistent with that found in series including only suspected adult MAS. [10]

Other series have noted an older age in patients with MAS. Thus, in the study by Fardet et al (median age=51 years) and in the study by Debaugnies (median age=59 years) [5,11].

In addition, two Tunisian studies of four and eleven cases of secondary MAS in adults respectively found median ages of 34.75 and 47.3 years. [12,13]

These observed differences can be explained by sampling fluctuations.

Etiologies

Infectious origin of MAS was the most frequent (54%) followed by systemic diseases (21%) and neoplasia (13%).

This is supported by the literature: viral causes are the most frequent among infections [14,15].

In our study, EBV, CMV and HIV were the most common viruses involved.

Among the bacterial causes, tuberculosis was the most frequent in our series given its endemic character in our country. In a systematic review of the literature, Ramos-Casals et al, stated that tuberculosis was responsible for MAS in 38% of cases [16].

In our series, only 3 patients had a haematological malignancy complicated by MAS. Higher prevalences have been reported in larger studies or in oncological settings [17].

A recent series found haematological malignancy as a causative factor for MAS in 92 of 162 cases (57%). Non-Hodgkin's Malignant Lymphoma (NHL) accounted for the largest proportion of these haemopathies (35%), but there was also a notable proportion of Hodgkin's disease (10.5%) and Castleman's disease (10.5%). Untransformed low-grade haemopathies are usually not accompanied by MAS [18].

More than 30 autoimmune diseases are associated with MAS, two of which are closely related: SLE and adult Still's disease. More cases of SLE associated with MAS than cases complicating adult Still's disease have been reported in the literature (133 vs 54, respectively), but the prevalence of MAS is higher in adult Still's disease [19]. In our series, one patient had SLE, one had adult Still's disease and one had PAN.

In the literature, 18% of MAS are labelled idiopathic [20]. In our series, no etiology was found in two patients after exhaustive etiological investigation (8.33%).

II- Impact of clinical parameters in the diagnosis of MAS :

Clinical symptoms in MAS are aspecific and occur acutely or subacutely. The cardinal signs are high fever (>38.5°C) and organomegaly. A quarter of patients may also show non-specific skin signs (erythematous rash, purpura, petechiae, etc.) or neurological signs such as coma, epileptic seizures, meningoencephalitis or meningeal haemorrhage. Digestive signs are observed in 18% of cases (diarrhoea, vomiting, abdominal pain) [14,15].

Constitutional or acquired immunosuppression status, known to favour the occurrence of haemophagocytosis, was present in 63% of cases in our work and in 30-60% in the literature series. This criterion is part of the diagnostic criteria retained by Fardet et al and included in the H-Score[5].

Fever, a cardinal sign of MAS. It is induced by different pro-inflammatory cytokines such as TNF-α, Il-1, Il-6 and IFN-gamma [15,21].

Its prevalence exceeds 90% in subjects with MAS in different studies, regardless of the underlying pathology. A systematic review of the literature conducted in 2018 identified 14 studies of MAS secondary to autoimmune diseases. In 10 studies, all patients were febrile [22]. Our results are consistent with those of the literature. Indeed, in our study, fever was the only clinical sign that distinguished the two groups (p=0.006).

Organomegaly is a characteristic clinical sign of MAS. Hepatosplenomegaly is secondary to infiltration of these organs by benign lymphohistiocytic proliferation [23]. In the literature, the prevalence of the observation of splenomegaly or hepatomegaly is variable (respectively 11% to 91.7% [24, 25] and 18% to 92.3% [24, 26]. Two major reviews of the literature were conducted by Karras et al in 2002 and Ramo-Casals et al in 2014 and included 306 and 775 patients respectively. The prevalence of splenomegaly was 42.8% and 69% respectively. That of hepatomegaly was 44.8% and 67% respectively [16,20]. However, although they are sensitive, these signs lack specificity and cannot be discriminatory. Our results are in agreement with the literature.

Cutaneous, respiratory and neurological manifestations are less common in MAS [27]. They may be secondary to MAS or to the underlying disease. In our study, these manifestations were not predictive of the diagnosis of MAS.

III-Impact of biological parameters in diagnostic orientation :

The biological abnormalities observed in MAS are numerous but non-specific. It is their association with clinical signs that leads to the diagnosis of MAS [16].

Cytopenias :

The presence of cytopenias on the blood count is a key feature of the clinico-biological presentation of MAS. Bicytopenia (typically thrombocytopenia and anaemia) is seen in up to 80% of adult cases and leukopenia in 69% [4]. Monocytopenia is less suggestive.

These cytopenias are secondary to intramedullary phagocytosis of haematopoietic elements but also secondary to depletion of myeloid precursors, reflecting the suppressive action of various pro-inflammatory cytokines such as TNF, Il-6 and IFN-gamma [28,29].

Thrombocytopenia is the earliest and most common blood count abnormality, with a central but sometimes peripheral mechanism, due to DIC.

In our study, ¾ of the patients in the "SAM group" were thrombocytopenic with a median value of 75000/mm3. Similar data have also been found in the literature [16,30].

Anemia in MAS is central, normochromic, with stigmata of intra-tissue haemolysis. In the study by Fradet et al, the threshold haemoglobin level adopted by the H-score is ≤9.2g/dL [5]. In our series, although the median haemoglobin level was 6.85 g/dL, it was not a discriminating factor between the two groups.

Leukopenia is less common and occurs later than other cytopenias. It is mainly characterised by neutropenia [26]. In our study, 54% of MAS patients were leukopenic. These results are close to those of the study by Ramos-Casals et al, (69%) [16].

However, neutropenia was less frequently observed in our patients.

Our results underline the importance of haematological involvement in MAS, although no significant difference was found between the two groups. This can be explained, on the one hand, by the low power of the study and, on the other hand, by the fact that febrile cytopenias are the main reason for suspicion of MAS in our study.

Ferritinemia :

90% of patients with MAS have hyperferritinemia, sometimes with extremely high levels [31]. The mechanisms of hyperferritinemia are multiple, involving excess excretion by macrophages, release during erythrophagocytosis and impaired clearance. Elevated ferritin levels are included in the HLH-2004 (>500 ng/mL) and HScore (>2000 ng/mL) criteria for the positive diagnosis of MAS. More recently, a threshold of 4420 ng/mL was used by Karikike et al for the diagnosis of MAS secondary to infections with a specificity of 97.1% and a PPV of 98% [4,5,32].

In our study, serum ferritin was a discriminating factor between the two groups (AUC=0.81; p=0.04), which is in line with all the data in the literature.

In addition, the collapse of the glycosylated fraction of ferritin has been proposed by some authors as a marker of severe MAS, but is not part of the diagnostic criteria recognised by the learned societies. [33].

Triglyceridemia :

Hypertriglyceridaemia is observed in up to 69% of MAS. It reflects the inhibition of lipoprotein lipase by high levels of TNFα [16]. In the H-score, the number of points attributed to this parameter is very important according to its value, which reflects the intensity of the association with the positive diagnosis [5].   Also, in our study, hypertriglyceridaemia was a highly discriminating parameter between the two groups (AUC= 0.88; *p=10-3*).

Hyponatremia

In MAS, hyponatremia is common. It is thought to be related to the syndrome of inappropriate ADH secretion.

In our series, we were able to demonstrate an association between the diagnosis of MAS and hyponatremia with good discriminatory power (AUC= 0.82; p=0.02). In both the H score and the HLH 2004, hyponatraemia was not considered a diagnostic criterion [5].

IV- Contribution of the myelogram study in the diagnosis of MAS: interest of the research of new cytological parameters

The myelogram is the cytological examination of choice for the detection of haemophagocytosis, which is found in approximately 84% of cases of MAS [16].

These images may be absent in the initial stages of the disease, so that some authors suggest that a repeat myelogram should be performed if the diagnosis is strongly suspected [34]. Conversely, the presence of haemophagocytosis images can be observed in severe septic states, the management of which is radically different from that of MAS [28].

Thus, making a diagnosis of MAS based on the presence of haemophagocytosis images is sometimes problematic.

In this regard, we performed a first reading of the marrow smears: a diagnostic reading that mainly assessed the richness of the marrow, the presence of macrophages and the presence of haemophagocytosis images.

The marrow richness was comparable in both the MAS and non-ASM groups. This is an expected result as it is accepted that the marrow smear in MAS is rich. This richness is also observed in reactive and inflammatory marrow.

In our study, only the presence of macrophages was associated with the diagnosis of MAS ($p=0.02$).

At the second reading of bone marrow smears, we sought to identify cytological criteria that would optimise referral for the diagnosis of adult MAS.

We studied the richness of the marrow in macrophages. Early publications suggested threshold macrophage infiltration rates of >3% marrow macrophages for Tsuda et al [35] and >2% macrophages for Wong et al [36], and these thresholds have been incorporated into diagnostic criteria for MAS. However, their successor diagnostic scores did not include macrophage richness as a criterion. In our study, the number of macrophages per 1000 nuclei was higher in MAS smears but the association with diagnosis was not demonstrated. This could be explained by the low power of the study on the one hand and by the excess of macrophages classically observed in reaction marrows on the other.

We also looked for an association between the intensity of haemophagocytosis and the positive diagnosis of MAS. Although intense marrow infiltration with haemophagocytosis images was only observed in the MAS group, no statistically significant association was found. This result could be explained by the small size of the two groups. Similar results were found in a recent study where an optimal threshold for the number of marrow HPCs could reliably distinguish patients in the low and high probability MAS categories [37].

In another study, the sensitivity of haemophagocytosis was 83% with a specificity of only 60%. The authors suggest that an increase in the threshold for haemophagocytosis from 0.05% to 0.13% would increase the specificity to 100% [7].

Furthermore, Iqbel et al studied the myelograms of 250 adult patients with MAS secondary to different etiologies. The intensity of haemophagocytosis was studied. The authors found that 35.50% of MAS were Grade I, 45.50% were Grade II, and 19.60% were Grade III. They also found that Grade III intensity was associated with cytopenias including anaemia and thrombocytopenia [38].

In relation to the aetiology of MAS, the intensity of haemophagocytosis has been found to be more frequent in MAS secondary to viral infection. It appears to be independent of marrow richness.

In addition, we sought to show the correspondence between the intensity of haemophagocytosis and the presence of cytopenias. The low power of the study largely explains the lack of association found. This finding was also noted by Strauss et al. The authors believe that the pathophysiological basis for the development of cytopenias is not solely based on the phagocytosis of marrow elements, but has multiple causes involving the aetiology of MAS and the degree of cytokine stimulation, particularly that of INF-gamma [39].

Using multiple logistic regression, we built several models incorporating the classical clinico-biological parameters introduced in the diagnostic criteria, but also cytological study criteria. The predictive abilities of all models were moderate. The contribution of the new cytological criteria did not seem to improve the quality of the equations.

At the end of this analysis, however, we would like to make a few comments:

Firstly, and more importantly, in the absence of any real contribution, a medullary study of 1000 nucleated elements, which can be long and tedious, clashes with the urgent nature of the myelogram result.

Secondly, in view of the results, we agree with the call for guidelines for bone marrow assessment in patients with clinico-biological signs of suspected MAS. It is particularly important for adults with secondary MAS because of the paucity of published studies on this subject [6,7].

CONCLUSION

Macrophage activation syndrome (MAS) is a rare clinical, biological and cytological entity that can be life-threatening. The condition is characterised by excessive and inappropriate activation of macrophages and the lymphoid system resulting in uncontrolled haemophagocytosis.

The exact prevalence of secondary MAS in adults remains unknown due to the difficulty in making a positive diagnosis. Indeed, MAS presents a polymorphous clinical picture most often associating fever and hepatosplenomegaly. From a biological point of view, no specific test is available. Nowadays, the association of cytopenias, hyperferritinemia and hypertriglyceridemia is suggestive of the diagnosis and the indication of a myelogram in search of images of haemophagocytosis is often given. However, the observation of haemophagocytosis is not specific to MAS.

Few publications have addressed the qualitative study of the myelogram and the cyto-morphological features observed in this disease. Furthermore, at the present time, there is no consensus on the number of threshold images to be observed or on the type of phagocytic cells to be observed in order to increase the sensitivity of the cytological study.

The main objective of our study was to determine the role of a more accurate reading of bone marrow smears through the search for cytological criteria to optimise the orientation towards the diagnosis of MAS in adults.

The clinical and biological data of our study population were largely consistent with those reported in the literature. The parameters associated with the diagnosis of MAS were fever, ferritinemia, triglyceridemia and LDH (respectively, p= 0.007, p= 0.04, p= 0.000, p= 0.034). In contrast, none of the cytological parameters studied were associated with the diagnosis. This corroborates the data in the literature. In addition, we performed a multiple regression study incorporating clinical-biological parameters classically introduced in the diagnostic criteria, but also criteria from the cytological study. The three models established had average predictive abilities for the positive diagnosis. The contribution of the new cytological criteria did not seem to improve the quality of the equations.

Thus, given the lack of real contribution, a bone marrow study of 1000 nucleated elements, which can be long and tedious, clashes with the urgent nature of the myelogram result. Nevertheless, guidelines for bone marrow assessment in patients with clinico-biological signs of suspected MAS remain to be defined.

REFERENCES

1- Brisse E, Wouters CH, Matthys P. Advances in the pathogenesis of primary and secondary haemophagocytic lymphohistiocytosis: Differences and similarities. *Br J Haematol.* 2016;174(2):203-17.

2- Hayden A, Park S, Giustini D, Lee AYY, Chen L. Hemophagocytic syndromes (HPSs) including hemophagocytic lymphohistiocytosis (HLH) in adults: a systematic scoping review. *Blood Rev* 2016;30:411-20

3- Tamamyan GN, Kantarjian HM, Ning J, Jain P, Sasaki K, Mcclain KL, Allen CE, Pierce SA, Cortes JE, Ravandi F, Konopleva MY, Garcia-Manero G, Benton CB, Chihara D, Rytting ME, Wang S, Abdelall W, Konoplev SN, Daver NG. Malignancy-associated hemophagocytic lymphohistiocytosis in adults: relation to hemophagocytosis, characteristics, and outcomes. *Cancer.* 2016;122:2857–66.

4- Henter JI, Horne A, Arico M, Egeler RM, Filipovich AH, Imashuku S, et al. HLH-2004: Diagnostic and therapeutic guidelines for hemophagocytic lymphohistiocytosis. *Pediatr Blood Cancer.*2007;48:124-131

5- Fardet L, Galicier L, Lambotte O, Marzac C, Aumont C, Chahwan D, et al. Development and validation of the hscore, a score for the diagnosis of reactive hemophagocytic syndrome. *Arthritis Rheumatol.* 2014;66(9):2613-20.

6- Ho C, Yao X, Tian L, Li FY, Podoltsev N, Xu ML. Marrow assessment for hemophagocytic lymphohistiocytosis demonstrates poor correlation with disease probability. *Am J Clin Pathol.* 2014;141(1):62-71.

7- Goel S, Polski JM, Imran H. Sensitivity and specificity of bone marrow hemophagocytosis in hemophagocytic lymphohistiocytosis. *Ann Clin Lab Sci.* 2012;42(1):21-5.

8- Bode, S.F., Lehmberg, K., Maul-Pavicic, A. *et al.* Recent advances in the diagnosis and treatment of hemophagocytic lymphohistiocytosis. *Arthritis Res Ther 2012;***14,** 213

9- Batu ED, Erden A, Seyhoglu E, Kilic L, Buyukasik Y, Karadag O, et al. Assessment of the hscore for reactive haemophagocytic syndrome in patients with rheumatic diseases. *Scand J Rheumatol.* 2017;46(1):44-8.

10- Kaito K, Kobayashi M, Katayama T, Otsubo H, Ogasawara Y, Sekita T, Saeki A, Sakamoto M, Nishiwaki K, Masuoka H, Shimada T, Yoshida M, Hosoya T. Prognostic factors of hemophagocytic syndrome in adults: analysis of 34 cases. *Eur J Haematol.* 1997;59:247-253.

11- Debaugnies F, Mahadeb B, Ferster A, Meuleman N, Rozen L, Demulder A, et al. Performance of the h-score for diagnosis of hemophagocytic lymphohistiocytosis in adult and pediatric patients. *Am J Clin Pathol.* 2016;145(6):862-70.

12- Ben Dhaou Hmaidi B DF, Boussema F, Ketari Jammoussi S, Baili L, Kochbati S, Cherif O, Rokbani L. Macrophagic activation syndrome: A props of 4 observations. *Tun Med.* 2011;89:70-5.

13- Boukhris I RI, Chérif E, Azzabi S, Ben Hassine L, Kéchaou I, Kaouech Z, Kooli C, Khalfallah N. Macrophagic activation syndrome: A series of 11 Tunisian cases. *Tun Med.* 2014;92:663-8

14- Novotny F, Simonetta F, Samii K, Chalandon Y, Serratrice J. [reactive hemophagocytic syndrome]. *Rev Med Suisse.* 2017;13(579):1797-803

15- Carter SJ, Tattersall RS, Ramanan AV. Macrophage activation syndrome in adults: Recent advances in pathophysiology, diagnosis and treatment. *Rheumatology (Oxford).* 2019;58(1):5-17

16- Ramos-Casals M, Brito-Zeron P, Lopez-Guillermo A, Khamashta MA, Bosch X. Adult haemophagocytic syndrome. *Lancet.* 2014;383(9927):1503-16.

17- Schram AM, Berliner N. How i treat hemophagocytic lymphohistiocytosis in the adult patient. *Blood.* 2015;125(19):2908-14

18-   Rivière S, Galicier L, Coppo P, Marzac C, Aumont C, Lambotte O, et al. Reactive Hemophagocytic Syndrome in Adults: A Retrospective Analysis of 162 Patients. *Am J Med*. 2014 Nov;127(11):1118-25

19-   Créput C, Galicier L, Oksenhendler E, Azoulay E. Lymphohistiocytic activation syndrome: review of the literature, implications in intensive care. *Réanimation*. 2005;14(7):604-13.

20-   Karras A, Hermine O. Hemophagocytic syndrome]. *Rev Med Interne*. 2002;23(9):768-78.

21-   Henter JI, Elinder G, Soder O, Hansson M, Andersson B, Andersson U. Hypercytokinemia in familial hemophagocytic lymphohistiocytosis. *Blood*. 1991;78(11):2918-22.

22-   Lerkvaleekul B, Vilaiyuk S. Macrophage activation syndrome: Early diagnosis is key. *Open Access Rheumatol*. 2018;10:117-28.

23-   Borgia RE, Gerstein M, Levy DM, Silverman ED, Hiraki LT. Features, treatment, and outcomes of macrophage activation syndrome in childhood-onset systemic lupus erythematosus. *Arthritis Rheumatol*. 2018;70(4):616-24.

24-   Latino GA, Manlhiot C, Yeung RS, Chahal N, McCrindle BW. Macrophage activation syndrome in the acute phase of kawasaki disease. *J Pediatr Hematol Oncol*. 2010;32(7):527-31.

25-   Zeng HS, Xiong XY, Wei YD, Wang HW, Luo XP. Macrophage activation syndrome in 13 children with systemic-onset juvenile idiopathic arthritis. *World J Pediatr*. 2008;4(2):97-101.

26-   Gonzalez F, Vincent F, Cohen Y. Macrophagic activation syndrome of infectious origin: Etiologies and management. *Reanimation*. 2009;18(4):284-90.

27-   Schram AM, Comstock P, Campo M, Gorovets D, Mullally A, Bodio K, et al. Haemophagocytic lymphohistiocytosis in adults: A multicentre case series over 7 years. *Br J Haematol.* 2016;172(3):412-9.

28-   Castillo L, Carcillo J. Secondary hemophagocytic lymphohistiocytosis and severe sepsis/systemic inflammatory response syndrome/ multiorgan dysfunction syndrome/macrophage activation syndrome share common intermediate phenotypes on a spectrum of inflammation. *Pediatr Crit Care Med.* 2009;10:387-392.

29-   Creput C, Galicier L, Buyse S, Azoulay E. Understanding organ dysfunction in hemophagocytic lymphohistiocytosis. Intensive Care Med. 2008;34(7):1177-87

30-   Li J, Wang Q, Zheng W, et al. Hemophagocytic lymphohistiocytosis: Clinical analysis of 103 adult patients. Medicine (Baltimore) 2014;93:100-5.

31-   Switala JR, Hendricks M, Davidson A. Serum ferritin is a cost-effective laboratory marker for hemophagocytic lymphohistiocytosis in the developing world. *J Pediatr Hematol Oncol.* 2012 Apr;34(3):e89-92

32-   Karakike E, Giamarellos-Bourboulis EJ. Macrophage activation-like syndrome: A distinct entity leading to early death in sepsis. *Front Immunol.* 2019;10:55.

33-   Wang Z, Wang Y, Wang J, Feng C, Tian L, Wu L. Early diagnostic value of low percentage of glycosylated ferritin in secondary hemophagocytic lymphohistiocytosis. *Int J Hematol.* 2009 Nov;90(4):501-5

34-   Gupta A, Weitzman S, Abdelhaleem M. The role of hemophagocytosis in bone marrow aspirates in the diagnosis of hemophagocytic lymphohistiocytosis. *Pediatr Blood Cancer.* 2008 Feb;50(2):192-4

35-   Tsuda H. Hemophagocytic syndrome (hps) in children and adults. *Int J Hematol.* 1997;65(3):215-26.

36-   Wong KF, Chan JK. Reactive hemophagocytic syndrome--a clinicopathologic study of 40 patients in an oriental population. *Am J Med.* 1992;93(2):177-80.

37-   Machaczka M, Klimkowska M, Ho C, et al. Bone marrow assessment in the diagnosis of acquired hemophagocytic lymphohistiocytosis in adults. *Am J Clin Pathol* 2015; 143: 308-310

38-   Iqbal W, Alsalloom AA, Shehzad K, Mughal F, Rasheed Z. Hemophagocytic histiocytosis: A Clinicopathological correlation. *Int J Health Sci (Qassim).* 2017;11(1):1–7.

39-   Strauss R, Neureiter D, Westenburger B, Wehler M, Kirchner T, Hahn EG. Multifactorial risk analysis of bone marrow histiocytic hyperplasia with hemophagocytosis in critically ill medical patients - A postmortem clinicopathologic analysis. *Crit Care Med* 2004;32:1316-21.

ANNEXES

Annex 1

SAM SHEET

Surname: first name: age: sex: department of origin: hospital file number :

Attending physician :

Medical history:

Known immunosuppression (HIV or immunosuppressive therapy):

Surgical history:

Progressive condition :

Treatment in progress :

Clinical :

Maximum temperature :

Hepatomegaly: Splenomegaly: Adenopathy:

Skin manifestations:

Neurological manifestations : (confusion, coma...)

Pulmonary manifestations :

Biology :

Leukocytes: neutrophils: lymphocytes: monocytes :

Haemoglobin (not transfused): the lowest figure :

Platelets (not transfused): the lowest number :

Ferritinemia: (the highest number)

Triglyceridemia:(the highest number)

Fibrinogen: (the lowest number)

Natremia :

LDH :

SGOT: (the highest number)

SGPT: (the highest number)

Total bilirubin :

PAL :

Gamma GT :

CRP :

Possibility to complete with some parameters (works) :

> *Serum interleukin 2: (high)*
>
> *Soluble CD25: (high)* sign of T cell activation
>
> *Soluble CD163: (high)* sign of macrophage activation
>
> *Albumin levels :*
>
> *DDimer :*

CD25/ferritin ratio: if > 8.5: in favour of lymphomatous origin of MAS

Myelogram :

Richness of the marrow :

% macrophages+/-

Images of haemophagocytosis: yes no

> If yes, number of images/blade :
>
> Nature of the phagocytosed elements :

HSCORE :

Etiological assessment :

ECBU :

Blood culture :

Serologies (viral, parasitic, etc.) :

Culture of other biological fluids :

Chest X-ray:

Scanner :

BOM :

Other :

PROBABLE ETIOLOGY :

Clinico-biological evolution:

Parameters	7 days	30 days	3 months	6 months
	Clinics			
Temperature				
Hepatomegaly				
Splenomegaly				
Adenopathies				
Other				
	Biological			
Hemoglobin				
Leukocytes				
PNN				
Lymphocytes				
Monocytes				
Plaques				
Ferritinemia				
Triglyceridemia				
Fibrinogen				
Natraemia				
LDH				
SGOT (ASAT)				
SGPT (ALAT)				
Total bilirubin				
PAL				
Gamma GT				
CRP				
Albumin				
D-Dimer				
Other				

Image of haemophagocytosis

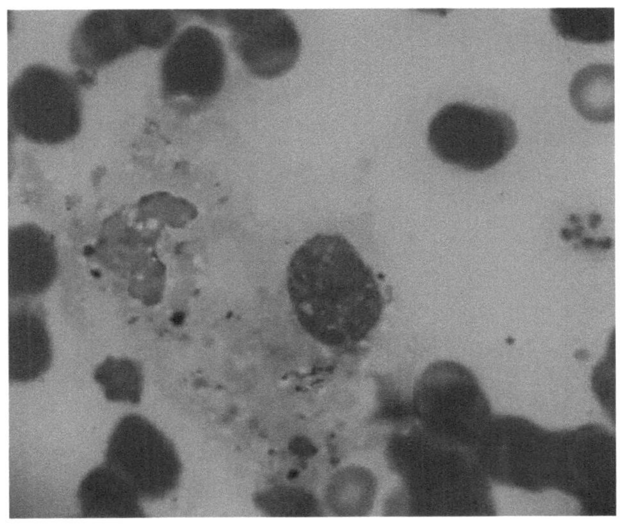

Image of multiple haemophagocytosis

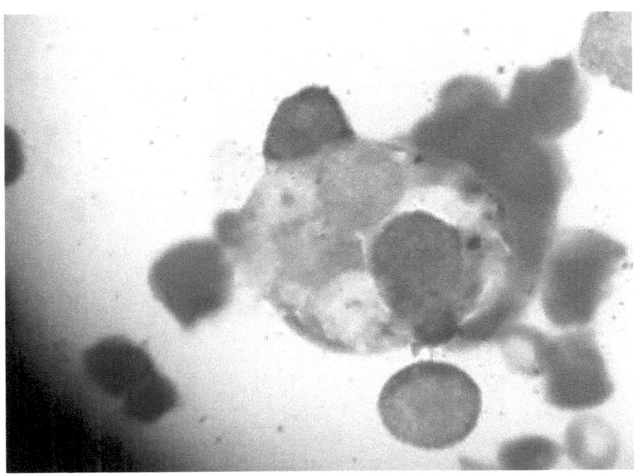

Annex 3:

Cytologiste : Dr Chakroun

FICHE CYTOLOGIQUE SAM

Méthodologie de lecture : sur le frottis de moelle le plus riche, on compte les macrophages, les images d'hémophagocytoses sur <u>1000 éléments nucléés</u>

Numéro de la lame :				
Richesse de la moelle : cotation en (+)				
Présence d'images d'hémophagocytose (oui /non)				
Nombre de Macrophages par **1000** éléments nucléés observés	éléments nucléés observés			
N=				
Nombre d'images d'hémophagocytose par **1000** éléments nucléés observés				
N=				
Éléments phagocytés observés	Hématies	Erythroblastes	Granuleux	plaquettes
Nature				
Nombre/ macrophage				
Images d'hémophagocytose multiple *oui/non* *(nbre et cellules phagocytées)*				

64

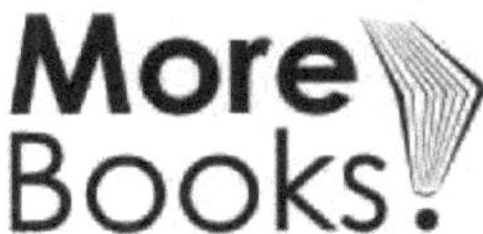

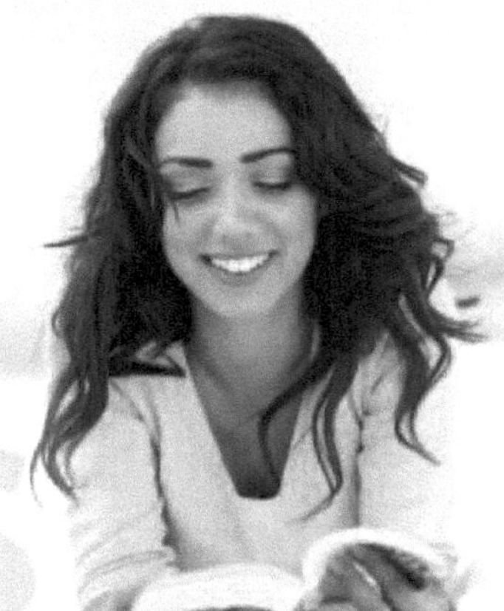

yes

I want morebooks!

Buy your books fast and straightforward online - at one of world's fastest growing online book stores! Environmentally sound due to Print-on-Demand technologies.

Buy your books online at
www.morebooks.shop

Kaufen Sie Ihre Bücher schnell und unkompliziert online – auf einer der am schnellsten wachsenden Buchhandelsplattformen weltweit! Dank Print-On-Demand umwelt- und ressourcenschonend produziert.

Bücher schneller online kaufen
www.morebooks.shop

KS OmniScriptum Publishing
Brivibas gatve 197
LV-1039 Riga, Latvia
Telefax: +371 686 204 55

info@omniscriptum.com
www.omniscriptum.com

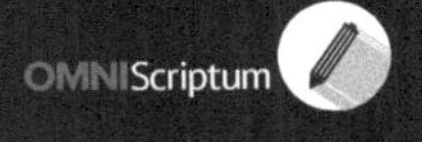